Anti-Inflammatory Diet Cookbook

The Ultimate Guide to Reduce Inflammation and Boost your Energy with Healthy and Budget-Friendly Recipes

Tiffany Chavez

Copyright 2021 - All rights reserved.

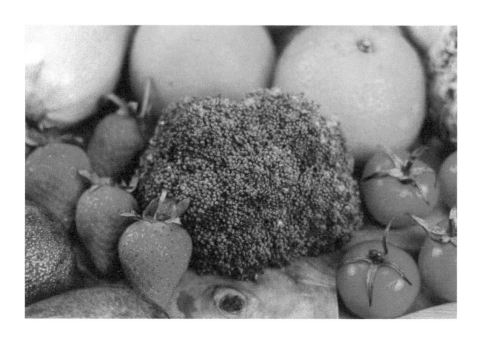

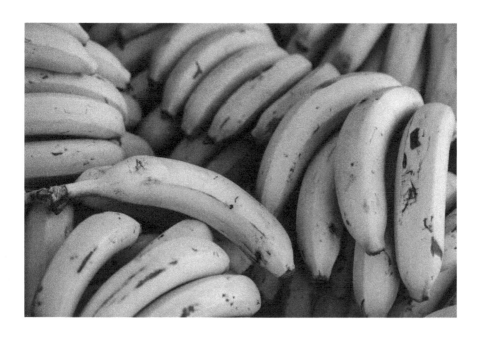

Table of Contents

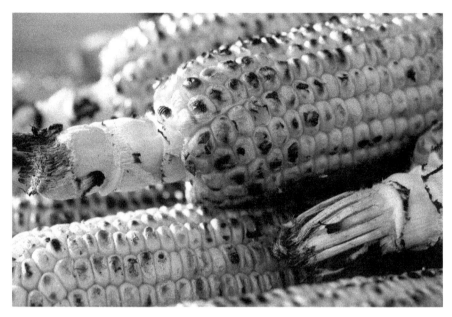

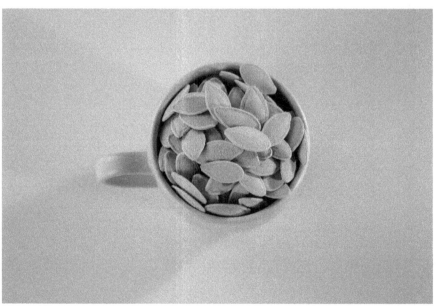

INTRODUCTION

An anti-inflammation diet entails eating only particular kinds of food and avoiding others to lower the symptoms of chronic inflammatory diseases. It is one of the recommended measures that an individual can take to reduce or prevent inflammation induced by diet.

Expectedly, an anti-inflammatory diet involves nutrient-dense plant foods and minimizing or avoiding processed meats and foods. The goal of an anti-inflammation diet is to minimize inflammatory responses. The diet entails substituting refined foods with whole and nutrient-laden foods. Predictably, an anti-inflammation diet will contain more amounts of antioxidants that are reactive molecules in food and help reduce the number of free radicals. The free radicals are molecules in the human body that may harm cells and enhance the risk of certain diseases.

Most of the widely consumed diets incorporate anti-inflammation diet principles. In particular, the Mediterranean diet has whole grains, fish, and fats that are beneficial for the heart. Studies suggest that this diet can help lower the effects of cardiovascular system inflammation due to diet. Taking an anti-inflammatory diet is can be a complementary therapy for most conditions that are aggravated by chronic inflammation.

Inflammation is a natural immune response, but it can also be triggered by outside forces such as allergies and autoimmune diseases. And when inflammation goes haywire, it can lead to all sorts of complications like heart disease, respiratory problems, premature aging, and even cancer.

That's why we're writing this blog post about how you can cure inflammation! You'll learn how it develops in the body and what triggers it so you can spot the warning signs before they escalate.

Inflammation is an important part of the immune system. When your body senses an intruder, it raises a red flag by releasing chemicals that travel to your lungs, heart, muscles, and skin. These chemical signals cause the cells that make up each tissue to release enzymes (cellular response regulators) that break down substances in the local area. This helps fight the threat without invading other parts of your body.

As an immune response, inflammation is a good thing. But if it's triggered by allergies or autoimmune diseases, your body can wind up attacking itself!

What are the signs of inflammation?

You may feel pain in your joints, swelling in the extremities like fingers and toes, and a general sense of feverishness. These symptoms are all signs of inflammation.

What causes inflammation?

As mentioned above, inflammation can be caused by outside factors like allergies or autoimmune diseases. But there are also triggers within the body itself that can set off an inflammatory response:

Oxygen shortage: Inadequate oxygen to the cells causes tissues to release too many chemicals that break down tissues and cause further problems. This can occur during high-intensity exercise and extreme situations such as heart attacks, strokes, and death.

Inadequate oxygen to the cells causes tissues to release too many chemicals that break down tissues and cause further problems. This can occur during high-intensity exercise and extreme situations such as heart attacks, strokes, and death.

Lack of nutrients: This is also known as oxidative stress. If cellular nutrients aren't getting to the cells, they will release chemicals to try and attract more nutrients. This can happen when cells become stressed or "old" (i.e. from excessive exposure to toxins), and the body can't produce enough energy to support them.

CHAPTER 1:

HOW TO CURE INFLAMMATION

Inflammation is a natural response to injury, and is usually thought of as being a boon to healing. But there are times when the immune system overreacts, causing too much inflammation which can be dangerous or even deadly.

Inflammation is a selective response to injury. It is thought of as being a boon to healing because of the rapid appearance of white blood cells, which are the body's first line of defense against bacteria and viruses. The purpose of inflammation is to fight infection, promote healing, and remove damaged tissue.

Due to an overload in the inflammatory pathways, a person may experience unwanted pain and discomfort. In addition, too much inflammation can damage healthy tissue along with infected or injured material, making it difficult to heal properly.

Chronic inflammation is the inflammatory response to any agent that continuously causes low-level inflammation because of systemic or chronic immune activation. This occurs when the body is unable to turn off the inflammatory response. Two common types of chronic inflammation include rheumatoid arthritis and osteoarthritis, though other types do exist.

A number of medications can directly cause immune system stimulation, causing excess inflammation. Some medications include: Corticosteroids, Lipitor, Metformin and Simvastatin can cause an increase in the inflammatory response which contributes to muscle aches and neuropathy symptoms. The use of vaccines and other immunizations can also increase the body's inflammatory response, causing signs of inflammation such as pain and joint stiffness. The common cold virus is also a cause for chronic inflammation because it can cause an immune system response that persists past the initial infection.

Chronic inflammation is linked to the development of several diseases including: rheumatoid arthritis, osteoarthritis, lupus, multiple sclerosis and even some forms of cancer. According to studies by professors at the University of Berkeley, a person with chronic inflammation is 74% more likely to develop rheumatoid arthritis than someone who doesn't have any symptoms.

The source of inflammation can be anything. For example, the common cold is often caused by a virus. Likewise, heartburn is caused by a substance in food or stomach acids. Inflammation can also be caused by stress, changes in hormones such as estrogen and testosterone, and from conditions such as gastritis, Crohn's disease and gastric ulcer.

Some diseases are linked to chronic inflammation but there are times when inflammation can be beneficial. For example: if bacteria infect the body it can cause inflammation which in turn helps to fight off the infection so that it does not become systemic and cause serious damage to do organs like the kidneys or lungs for example.

How to Cure Inflammation - There are several steps you can take to reduce inflammation from chronic conditions such as osteoarthritis, rheumatoid arthritis and other autoimmune diseases. Your first step should be to schedule an appointment with a physician. The physician will likely have you undergo a series of tests including blood work and body scans. A diagnosis will then be made that will determine the course of treatment that is most appropriate for your condition.

The first step in treating inflammation is to completely eliminate all alcohol consumption from your diet because alcohol is a very potent inflammatory agent. Alcohol causes less inflammation in one's body the first time it is consumed. However, the more alcohol that is consumed, the greater chance there is for chronic inflammation to develop.

A diet that helps reduce inflammation begins with eliminating all processed sugars from the diet. Processed sugar depletes your body of antioxidants which are needed to fight off infection and disease, and it contributes to stress levels in your body because your body has a tough time breaking down all of that sugar. The ideal daily intake of sugar should be no more than 30 grams. A high protein intake along with a balanced amount of fats and complex carbohydrates will help to regulate hormones and blood sugar levels, which can have a positive impact on reducing inflammation in the body.

A healthy diet can also help to reduce inflammation by ensuring that you get enough vitamins and minerals to maintain a healthy immune system. For example, research has shown that people with chronic conditions such as rheumatoid arthritis were more likely to have varicose veins and high cholesterol levels when their dietary habits involved a lot of processed foods.

Fiber is a crucial nutrient for your body because it helps to move waste throughout the body, while also preventing constipation. Unfortunately, many Americans don't get enough fiber in their diet. Your body needs 20-30 grams of fiber per day. A good source of fiber will be vegetables with each serving containing at least 5 grams of fiber. You can also increase fiber in your diet by eating more whole grains, beans and legumes.

Reducing inflammation is not just about diet. It is also possible to tone down the inflammatory response in your body by modulating the way you look. By improving your fitness levels and strength, you will be able to exert yourself with less pain and discomfort which can help reduce inflammation.

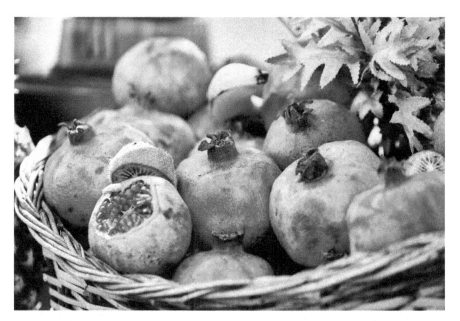

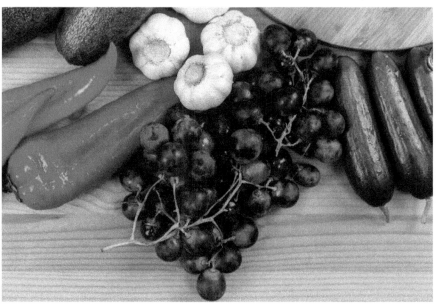

CHAPTER 2:

BREAKFAST

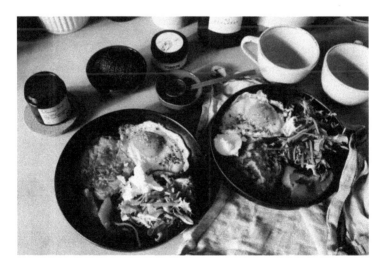

1. <u>White and Green Quiche</u>

Difficulty level: Easy

Preparation time: 10 minutes

Cooking Time: 40 minutes

Servings: 3

Ingredients:

- 3 cups of fresh spinach, chopped

- 15 large free-range eggs

- 3 cloves of garlic, minced

- 5 white mushrooms, sliced

- 1 small sized onion, finely chopped

- 1 ½ teaspoon of baking powder

- Ground black pepper to taste

- 1 ½ cups of coconut milk

- Ghee, as required to grease the dish

- Sea salt to taste

Directions:

1. Set the oven to 350°F.

2. Get a baking dish then grease it with the organic ghee.

3. Break all the eggs in a huge bowl then whisk well. Stir in coconut milk. Beat well

4. While you are whisking the eggs, start adding the remaining ingredients in it.

5. When all the ingredients are thoroughly blended, pour all of it into the prepared baking dish. Bake for at least 40 minutes, up to the quiche is set in the middle. Enjoy!

Nutrition: Calories: 608 kcal Protein: 20.28 g Fat: 53.42 g Carbohydrates: 16.88 g

2. <u>**Beef Breakfast Casserole**</u>

Difficulty level: Easy

Preparation time: 10 minutes

Cooking Time: 30 minutes

Servings: 5

Ingredients:

- 1 pound of ground beef, cooked

- 10 eggs

- ½ cup Pico de Gallo

- 1 cup baby spinach

- ¼ cup sliced black olives

- Freshly ground black pepper

Directions:

1. Preheat oven to 350 degrees Fahrenheit. Prepare a 9" glass pie plate with non-stick spray.

2. Whisk the eggs until frothy. Season with salt and pepper.

3. Layer the cooked ground beef, Pico de Gallo, and spinach in the pie plate.

4. Slowly pour the eggs over the top.

5. Top with black olives.

6. Bake for at least 30 minutes, until firm in the middle.

7. Slice into 5 pieces and serve.

Nutrition: Calories: 479 kcal Protein: 43.54 g Fat: 30.59 g Carbohydrates: 4.65 g

3. **Ham and Veggie Frittata Muffins**

Difficulty level: Easy

Preparation time: 10 minutes

Cooking Time: 25 minutes

Servings: 12

Ingredients:

- 5 ounces thinly sliced ham

- 8 large eggs

- 4 tablespoons coconut oil

- ½ yellow onion, finely diced

- 8 oz. frozen spinach, thawed and drained

- 8 oz. mushrooms, thinly sliced

- 1 cup cherry tomatoes, halved

- ¼ cup coconut milk (canned)

- 2 tablespoons coconut flour

- Sea salt and pepper to taste

Directions:

1. Preheat oven to 375 degrees Fahrenheit.

2. In a medium skillet, warm the coconut oil on medium heat. Add the onion and cook until softened.

3. Add the mushrooms, spinach, and cherry tomatoes. Season with salt and pepper. Cook until the mushrooms have softened. About 5 minutes. Remove from heat and set aside.

4. In a huge bowl, beat the eggs together with the coconut milk and coconut flour. Stir in the cooled the veggie mixture.

5. Line each cavity of a 12 cavity muffin tin with the thinly sliced ham. Pour the egg mixture into each one and bake for 20 minutes.

6. Remove from oven and allow to cool for about 5 minutes before transferring to a wire rack.

7. To maximize the benefit of a vegetable-rich diet, it's important to eat a variety of colors, and these veggie-packed frittata muffins do just that. The onion, spinach, mushrooms, and cherry tomatoes provide a wide range of vitamins and nutrients and a healthy dose of fiber.

Nutrition: Calories: 125 kcal Protein: 5.96 g Fat: 9.84 g Carbohydrates: 4.48 g

4. <u>Tomato and Avocado Omelet</u>

Difficulty level: Easy

Preparation time: 5 minutes

Cooking Time: 5 minutes

Servings: 1

Ingredients:

- 2 eggs

- ¼ avocado, diced

- 4 cherry tomatoes, halved

- 1 tablespoon cilantro, chopped

- Squeeze of lime juice

- Pinch of salt

Directions:

1. Put together the avocado, tomatoes, cilantro, lime juice, and salt in a small bowl, then mix well and set aside.

2. Warm a medium nonstick skillet on medium heat. Whisk the eggs until frothy and add to the pan. Move the eggs around gently with a rubber spatula until they begin to set.

3. Scatter the avocado mixture over half of the omelet. Remove from heat, and slide the omelet onto a plate as you fold it in half.

4. Serve immediately.

Nutrition: Calories: 433 kcal Protein: 25.55 g Fat: 32.75 g Carbohydrates: 10.06 g

5. Vegan-Friendly Banana Bread

Difficulty level: Easy

Preparation time: 15 minutes

Cooking Time: 40 minutes

Servings: 4-6

Ingredients:

- 2 ripe bananas, mashed

- 1/3 cup brewed coffee

- 3 tbsp. chia seeds

- 6 tbsp. water

- ½ cup soft vegan butter

- ½ cup maple syrup

- 2 cups flour

- 2 tsp. baking powder

- 1 tsp. cinnamon powder

- 1 tsp. allspice

- ½ tsp. salt

Directions:

1. Set oven at 350F.

2. Bring the chia seeds in a small bowl then soak it with 6 tbsp. of water. Stir well and set aside.

3. In a mixing bowl, mix using a hand mixer the vegan butter and maple syrup until it turns fluffy. Add the chia seeds along with the mashed bananas.

4. Mix well and then add the coffee.

5. Meanwhile, sift all the dry ingredients (flour, baking powder, cinnamon powder, all spice, and salt) and then gradually add into the bowl with the wet ingredients.

6. Combine the ingredients well and then pour over a baking pan lined with parchment paper.

7. Place in the oven to bake for at least 30-40 minutes, or until the toothpick comes out clean after inserting in the bread.

8. Allow the bread to cool before serving.

Nutrition: Calories: 371 kcal Protein: 5.59 g Fat: 16.81 g Carbohydrates: 49.98 g

6. <u>**Mango Granola**</u>

Difficulty level: Easy

Preparation time: 10 minutes

Cooking Time: 30 minutes

Servings: 4

Ingredients:

- 2 cups rolled oats

- 1 cup dried mango, chopped

- ½ cup almonds, roughly chopped

- ½ cup nuts

- ½ cup dates, roughly chopped

- 3 tbsp. sesame seeds

- 2 tsp. cinnamon

- 2/3 cup agave nectar

- 2 tbsp. coconut oil

- 2 tbsp. water

Directions:

1. Set oven at 320F

2. In a large bowl, put the oats, almonds, nuts, sesame seeds, dates, and cinnamon then mix well.

3. Meanwhile, heat a saucepan over medium heat, pour in the agave syrup, coconut oil, and water.

4. Stir and let it cook for at least 3 minutes or until the coconut oil has melted.

5. Gradually pour the syrup mixture into the bowl with the oats and nuts and stir well, ensure that all the ingredients are coated with the syrup.

6. Transfer the granola on a baking sheet lined with parchment paper and place in the oven to bake for 20 minutes.

7. After 20 minutes, take off the tray from the oven and lay the chopped dried mango on top. Put back in the oven then bake again for another 5 minutes.

8. Let the granola cool to room temperature before serving or placing it in an airtight container for storage. The shelf life of the granola will last up to 2-3 weeks.

Nutrition: Calories: 434 kcal Protein: 13.16 g Fat: 28.3 g Carbohydrates: 55.19 g

7. <u>**Sautéed Veggies on Hot Bagels**</u>

Difficulty level: Medium

Preparation time: 10 minutes

Cooking Time: 16 minutes

Servings: 2

Ingredients:

- 1 yellow squash, diced

- 1 zucchini, sliced thin

- ½ onion, sliced thin

- 2 pcs. tomatoes, sliced

- 1 clove of garlic, chopped

- salt and pepper to taste

- 1 tbsp. olive oil

- 2 pcs. vegan bagels

- vegan butter for spread

Directions:

1. Heat the olive oil on the medium temperature in a cast-iron skillet.

2. Lower the heat to medium-low and sauté the onions for 10 minutes or until the onions start to brown.

3. Turn the heat again to medium and then add the diced squash and zucchini to the pan and cook for 5 minutes. Add the clove of garlic and cook for another minute.

4. Throw in the tomato slices to the pan and cook for 1 minute. Season with pepper and salt and turn off the heat.

5. Toast the bagels and cut in half.

6. Spread the bagels lightly with butter and serve with the sautéed veggies on top.

Nutrition: Calories: 375 kcal Protein: 14.69 g Fat: 11.46 g Carbohydrates: 54.61 g

8. <u>Coco-Tapioca Bowl</u>

Difficulty level: Medium Preparation time: 10 minutes

Cooking Time: 20 minutes Servings: 2

Ingredients:

- ¼ cup tapioca pearls, small sized

- 1 can light coconut milk ¼ cup maple syrup

- 1 ½ tsp. lemon juice

- ½ cup unsweetened coconut flakes, toasted

- 2 cups water

Directions:

1. Place the tapioca in a saucepan and pour over the 2 cups of water. Let it stand for at least 30 minutes.

2. Pour in the coconut milk and syrup and heat the saucepan over medium temperature. Bring to a boil while stirring constantly.

3. Add the lemon juice and stir and then garnish with coconut flakes.

Nutrition: Calories: 309 kcal Protein: 3.93 g Fat: 9.02 g Carbohydrates: 54.55 g

9. Choco-Banana Oats

Difficulty level: Medium Preparation time: 5 minutes

Cooking Time: 8 minutes Servings: 2

Ingredients:

- 2 cups oats

- 2 cups almond milk

- ¾ cup water

- 2 ripe bananas, sliced

- ¼ tsp. Vanilla

- ¼ tsp. almond extract

- 2 tbsp. cocoa powder, unsweetened

- 2 tbsp. agave nectar

- 1/8 tsp. cinnamon 1/8 tsp. salt

- 1/3 cup toasted walnuts, chopped

- 2 tbsp. vegan chocolate chips, semisweet

Directions:

1. In a large saucepan, pour the almond milk, water, bananas, vanilla, and almond extract. Add the salt, stir, and heat over high temperature.

2. Mix the oats in the pan along with the unsweetened cocoa powder, 1 tbsp. agave nectar and lower the temperature to medium. Cook for 7-8 minutes, or until the oats are cooked to your liking. Stir frequently.

3. Scoop the cooked oats into serving bowls and garnish with the chopped walnuts, chocolate chips, and drizzle with the remaining agave nectar.

Nutrition: Calories: 522 kcal Protein: 30.17 g Fat: 27.01 g Carbohydrates: 79.09 g

10. <u>Savory Bread</u>

Difficulty level: Medium

Preparation time: 10 minutes

Cooking Time: 20-25 minutes

Servings: 8-10

Ingredients:

- ½ cup plus 1tablespoon almond flour

- 1 tsp. baking soda

- 1 teaspoon ground turmeric

- Salt, to taste

- 2 large organic eggs

- 2 organic egg whites

- 1 cup raw cashew butter

- 1 tablespoon water

- 1 tablespoon apple cider vinegar

Directions:

1. Set the oven to 350F. Grease a loaf pan.

2. In a big pan, mix together flour, baking soda, turmeric, and salt.

3. In another bowl, add eggs, egg whites, and cashew butter and beat till smooth.

4. Gradually, add water and beat till well combined.

5. Add flour mixture and mix till well combined.

6. Stir in apple cider vinegar treatment.

7. Place a combination into prepared loaf pan evenly.

8. Bake for around twenty minutes or till a toothpick inserted within the center is released clean.

Nutrition: Calories: 347 Fat: 11g Carbohydrates: 29g Fiber: 6g Protein: 21g

11. <u>**Savory Veggie Muffins**</u>

Difficulty level: Medium

Preparation time: 15 minutes

Cooking Time: 18-23 minutes

Servings: 5

Ingredients:

- ¾ cup almond meal

- ½ tsp baking soda

- ¼ cup concentrate powder

- 2 teaspoons fresh dill, chopped

- Salt, to taste

- 4 large organic eggs

- 1½ tablespoons nutritional yeast

- 2 teaspoons apple cider vinegar

- 3 tablespoons fresh lemon juice

- 2 tablespoons coconut oil, melted

- 1 cup coconut butter, softened

- 1 bunch scallion, chopped

- 2 medium carrots, peeled and grated

- ½ cup fresh parsley, chopped

Directions:

1. Set the oven to 350F. Grease 10 cups of your large muffin tin.

2. In a large bowl, mix together flour, baking soda, Protein powder, and salt.

3. In another bowl, add eggs, nutritional yeast, vinegar, lemon juice, and oil and beat till well combined.

4. Add coconut butter and beat till the mixture becomes smooth.

5. Put egg mixture into the flour mixture and mix till well combined.

6. Fold in scallion, carts, and parsley.

7. Place the amalgamation into prepared muffin cups evenly.

8. Bake for about 18-23 minutes or till a toothpick inserted inside center comes out clean.

Nutrition: Calories: 378 Fat: 13g Carbohydrates: 32g Fiber: 11g Protein: 32g

CHAPTER 3:

SEAFOOD

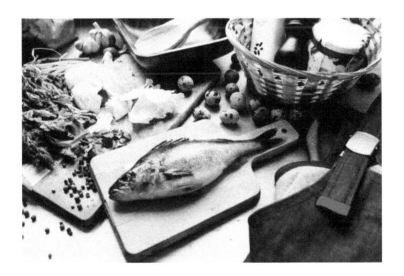

12. **Thai Chowder**

Difficulty level: Easy

Preparation time: 10 minutes

Cooking Time: 20 minutes

Servings: 6

Ingredients:

- 3 cups 98 % fat-free chicken broth

- 10 small red potatoes, diced

- 3 cobs fresh sweet corn

- 3/4 cup coconut milk

- 1/2 teaspoon fresh ginger, diced

- 1 teaspoon dried lemongrass

- 1 teaspoon green curry paste

- 1/2 cup cabbage, chopped

- Four 5-ounce tilapia fillets

- 2 tablespoons fish sauce

- 3/4 cup fresh shrimp, cleaned, with tails on

- 3/4 cup bay scallops

- 3/4 cup cilantro, chopped

Directions:

1. In a saucepan, boil chicken stock at high heat until it reaches a simmer. Decrease temperature and add the cabbage, ginger, coconut milk, lemongrass, sweet corn, and lemongrass, curry paste, and potatoes — cover and cook for 15 minutes.

2. Firstly, combine fish fillets and fish sauce, and cook for 6 minutes. Secondly, add the shrimp, and cook for a further 2 to 3 minutes. Finally, add the scallops and cook until scallops are opaque in color.

3. Serve with cilantro.

Nutrition: Calories: 761 kcal Protein: 33.25 g Fat: 5.34 g Carbohydrates: 150.45 g

13. **Tuna-Stuffed Tomatoes**

Difficulty level: Easy

Preparation time: 10 minutes

Cooking Time: 10 minutes

Servings: 2

Ingredients:

- 1 medium tomato

- 1 6oz. can tuna, drained and flaked

- 2 tbsp. mayonnaise

- 1 tbsp. celery, chopped

- ½ tsp. Dijon mustard

- ¼ tsp. seasoning salt

- Shredded mild cheddar cheese, to garnish

Directions:

1. Preheat oven to 375°. Wash tomato and cut in half from the stem. Using a tsp., scoop out tomato pulp and any seeds until you have two ½" shells remaining.

2. In a small mixing bowl, combine tuna, mayonnaise, celery, mustard, and seasoning salt. Stir until well blended.

3. Scoop an equal amount of tuna mixture into each ½ tomato shell. Place on a baking sheet and sprinkle shredded cheddar cheese over the top of each tuna-stuffed tomato shell. Bake for 7 to 8 minutes or until cheese is melted and golden-brown in color.

4. Serve immediately. Any remaining mixture can be safely stored, covered, in the fridge for up to 72 hours.

Nutrition: Calories: 175 kcal Protein: 21.24 g Fat: 8.79 g Carbohydrates: 3.04 g

14. <u>Seared Ahi Tuna</u>

Difficulty level: Easy

Preparation time: 10 minutes

Cooking Time: 15 minutes

Servings: 2

Ingredients:

- 2 (4-ounces each) ahi tuna steaks (3/4-inch thick)

- 2 tbsp. dark sesame oil

- 2 tbsp. soy sauce

- 1 tbsp. of grated fresh ginger

- 1 clove garlic, minced

- 1 green onion (scallion) thinly sliced, reserve a few slices for garnish

- 1 tsp. lime juice

Directions:

1. Begin by preparing the marinade. In a small bowl, put together the sesame oil, soy sauce, fresh ginger, minced garlic, green onion, and lime juice. Mix well.

2. Place tuna steaks into a sealable Ziploc freezer bag and pour marinade over the top of the tuna. Seal bag and shake or massage with hands to coat tuna steaks well with marinade. Bring the bag in a bowl, in case of breaks, and place tuna in the refrigerator to marinate for at least 10 minutes.

3. Place a large non-stick skillet over medium-high to high heat. Let the pan heat for 2 minutes, when hot, remove tuna steaks from the marinade and lay them in the pan to sear for 1-1½ minutes on each side.

4. Remove tuna steaks from pan and cut into ¼-inch thick slices. Garnish with a sprinkle of sliced green onion. Serve immediately.

Nutrition: Calories: 213 kcal Protein: 4.5 g Fat: 19.55 g Carbohydrates: 5.2 g

15. <u>**Bavette with Seafood**</u>

Difficulty level: Easy

Preparation time: 10 minutes

Cooking Time: 10 minutes

Servings: 4

Ingredients:

- Braised olive oil

- 200g clean medium shrimp

- 200g of clean octopus

- 200g mussel without shell

- 200g of clean squid cut into rings

- Salt to taste

- Black pepper to taste

- 1 clove minced garlic

- 400g peeled tomatoes

- 2 tablespoons coarse salt

- 350g of Bavette Barilla

- Chopped cilantro to taste

- ½ Lemon Juice

Directions:

1. In olive oil sauté the shrimp, the octopus, the mussel and the squid separately. Season with salt and black pepper.

2. In the same pan, sauté the garlic.

3. Add the peeled tomatoes, mix well — Cook for 2 minutes.

4. In a pan of boiling water, arrange 2 tablespoons of coarse salt and cook Bavette Barilla.

5. Remove Bavette Barilla 2 minutes before the time indicated on the package. Reserve the pasta cooking water if necessary.

6. Return the seafood to the sauce.

7. Arrange 1 scoop of the cooking water in the seafood sauce and add the drained pasta. Cook for another 2 minutes.

8. Finish with cilantro and lemon juice.

9. Serve immediately.

Nutrition: Calories: 526 kcal Protein: 40.59 g Fat: 24 g Carbohydrates: 38.02 g

16. **Quick Shrimp Moqueca**

Difficulty level: Easy

Preparation time: 10 minutes

Cooking Time: 10 minutes

Servings: 4

Ingredients:

- 600g Shrimp Peeled and Clean

- Salt to taste

- Juice of 2 lemons

- Braised olive oil

- 2 chopped purple onions

- 4 cloves garlic, minced

- 3 chopped tomatoes

- 1 chopped red pepper

- 1 chopped yellow pepper

- 1 cup tomato passata

- 200ml of coconut milk

- 2 finger peppers

- 2 tablespoons palm oil

- Chopped cilantro to taste

Directions:

1. In a container, arrange shrimp, season with salt and lemon juice and set aside.

2. In a hot pan, arrange olive oil and sauté onion and garlic.

3. Add the chopped tomatoes and sauté well.

4. Add the peppers and the tomato passata. Let it cook for a few minutes.

5. Add coconut milk, mix well.

6. Add the shrimp to the sauce.

7. Finally, add the finger pepper, palm oil, and chopped coriander.

8. Serve with rice and crumbs.

Nutrition: Calories: 426 kcal Protein: 46.15 g Fat: 15.46 g Carbohydrates: 26.26 g

17. **Fried ball of cod**

Difficulty level: Easy

Preparation time: 10 minutes

Cooking Time: 10 minutes

Servings: 4

Ingredients:

- Braised olive oil

- 1 red onion cut into strips

- 2 cloves garlic, minced

- 700g desalted and shredded cod

- ½ cup sliced black olive

- 3 minced boiled eggs

- Parsley to taste

- Salt to taste

- Black pepper

Directions:

1. In a hot skillet, arrange the olive oil and sauté the onion and then the garlic.

2. Add cod and sauté well.

3. Turn off the heat, then put the olives, the chopped eggs, and the parsley.

4. Correct salt if necessary, add pepper, and set aside to cool.

5. Stuff the pastry dough and close by brushing water and kneading with a fork.

6. Fry in hot oil by dipping until golden brown.

7. Drain on paper towels and serve.

Nutrition: Calories: 253 kcal Protein: 35.45 g Fat: 9.61 g Carbohydrates: 3.86 g

18. <u>Seafood Paella</u>

Difficulty level: Easy

Preparation time: 10 minutes

Cooking Time: 15 minutes

Servings: 2

Ingredients:

- Extra virgin olive oil

- 1 chopped onion

- 2 cloves minced garlic + 4 whole cloves garlic in shell

- ½ chopped green peppers

- ½ chopped yellow pepper

- ½ chopped red peppers

- 400g of the pump or parboiled rice

- 400g of sliced cooked octopus

- 400g squid in rings

- 2 packets of turmeric dissolved in 1.2 liters of fish stock

- Salt to taste

- Black pepper to taste

- 400g of pre-cooked shrimp

- 200g of frozen pea 500g mussel

- ½ packet of chopped parsley Chilies to decorate

- 4 units pre-cooked whole prawn

- Lemon juice

Directions:

1. In olive oil, sauté onion, garlic, peppers, and rice.

2. Add the octopus, the squid, and half the broth. Adjust salt and pepper.

3. As the liquid dries, add more broth taking care of the rice point.

4. When the stock is almost completely dry, add the shrimp and the pea.

5. Add the mussels and parsley.

6. Arrange peppers on top for garnish and prawns

7. Let it cook for 15 minutes with the pan covered.

8. Finish with lemon juice and olive oil.

Nutrition: Calories: 1468 kcal Protein: 177.19 g Fat: 28.65 g Carbohydrates: 115.89 g

19. **Vietnamese Roll and Tarê**

Difficulty level: Medium Preparation time: 20 minutes

Cooking Time: 10 minutes   Servings: 4

Ingredients:

- 1 cup of soy sauce

- 1 cup of sake baby

- 1 cup of sugar

- 6 sheets of rice paper

- Warm water

- Mint leaves

- 250g sauteed medium prawns

- 1 cup carrot cut into sticks

- 1 cup chopped Japanese cucumber

- 6 shredded lettuce leaves

- 1 ½ cup rice noodles prepared per package instructions

Directions:

1. Bring the soy sauce, sake, and sugar to medium heat. Stir from time to time and cook the mixture until it reduces to ⅓ of the

initial amount and obtain a soft syrup consistency. Set aside to cool.

2. Dip the rice leaf in warm water for about 30 seconds or until it softens.

3. Arrange on a flat surface and stuff the center of the rice paper with mint leaves, prawns, carrot, cucumber, lettuce, and pasta.

4. Roll up, cut in half and half again. Repeat the process with the other sheets of rice paper.

5. Serve with taré sauce.

Nutrition: Calories: 552 kcal Protein: 10.54 g Fat: 20.48 g Carbohydrates: 82.12 g

20. **Shrimp Pie**

Difficulty level: Medium

Preparation time: 15 minutes

Cooking Time: 35 minutes

Servings: 4-8

Ingredients:

- 250g of flour

- 200g of unsalted cold butter

- 1 teaspoon salt

- 3 tbsp. water

- 2 tbsp. olive oil

- 2 cloves garlic, minced

- 400g peeled clean shrimp

- 1 tomato without skin and without chopped seed

- 2 tbsp. coconut milk

- 1 minced finger pepper

- salt

- ¼ cup sour cream

- 2 tbsp. chopped cilantro

- 1 gem

Directions:

1. Place the flour in a bowl then add the diced butter.

2. Knead with fingertips until crumbly.

3. Add salt and, gradually, water until it turns into dough. Cover with plastic and refrigerate for 1 hour.

4. Heat a frying pan, sprinkle with olive oil and brown the garlic and prawns.

5. Add the tomatoes, sauté for a couple of minutes, then add coconut milk and pepper and cook for another two minutes.

6. Season with salt, add the cream, turn off the heat and add the cilantro. Set aside to cool.

7. To open the dough in portions and cover the pancakes, stuff with the shrimp, and cover with a circle of dough.

8. Brush with the yolk and bake in the preheated oven at 180 degrees for about 30 minutes or until golden brown.

Nutrition: Calories: 344 kcal Protein: 15.6 g Fat: 19.79 g Carbohydrates: 25.33 g

21. <u>**Seafood Noodles**</u>

Difficulty level: Medium

Preparation time: 10 minutes

Cooking Time: 20 minutes

Servings: 2

Ingredients:

- Braised olive oil

- 4 cloves garlic, minced

- 300g of clean squid cut into rings

- 200g mussel without shell

- 200g shell-less volley

- 10 clean prawns

- 150g of dried tomatoes

- salt to taste

- black pepper to taste

- 500g of pre-cooked noodles

- ½ pack of watercress

- ½ Lemon Juice

- parsley to taste

Directions:

1. In olive oil, sauté the garlic and add the squid, the mussel, the shrimp, and the shrimp.

2. Put the dried tomatoes and season with salt and pepper.

3. Add the noodles, watercress, season with lemon juice, and parsley.

Nutrition: Calories: 2049 kcal Protein: 56.21 g Fat: 143.36 g Carbohydrates: 139.98 g

22. **Potato Dumpling with Shrimp**

Difficulty level: Medium

Preparation time: 15 minutes

Cooking Time: 50 minutes

Servings: 6-8

Ingredients:

- 500g of pink potatoes

- 1 egg

- salt to taste

- 1 tbsp. chopped parsley

- 2 tablespoons flour + flour for handling and breading

- 10 units of clean giant tailed shrimp

- black pepper to taste

- ½ packet of chopped cilantro

- 3 tablespoons palm oil

- 4 lemon juice

- frying oil

Directions:

1. Put the potato to cook for 40 minutes.

2. When very tender, remove from heat, let cool and mash potatoes already peeled.

3. Add the egg and mix well, season with salt and parsley and add the flour. Set aside in the fridge for 2 hours.

4. Make small transverse cuts on the belly of the shrimp, without cutting to the end. Season the shrimp with black pepper, salt chopped coriander, palm oil, and lemon juice. Leave marinating for 15 minutes.

5. Take a portion of the potato flour dough in your hands and shape around a shrimp leaving the tail out.

6. Rinse flour again and fry in hot oil until golden.

Nutrition: Calories: 159 kcal Protein: 6.95 g Fat: 8.42 g Carbohydrates: 14.48 g

23. **Shrimp Rissoles**

Difficulty level: Medium

Preparation time: 10 minutes

Cooking Time: 30 minutes

Servings: 4

Ingredients:

- 1 tbsp. olive oil

- ½ diced onion

- 400g of shrimp

- 2 tbsp. tomato extract

- ½ packet of chopped parsley

- Salt to taste

- 250ml of water

- 250ml of milk

- 50g of butter

- 3 cups flour

- 100 g of curd

- 3 beaten eggs

- Breadcrumbs for breading

Directions:

1. Sauté with olive oil, onion, and shrimp.

2. Add tomato extract, parsley, and salt. Reserve.

3. In a pan, bring to medium heat water, milk and butter.

4. When the butter has melted, add 2 cups of wheat flour at a time and stir until the dough begins to unglue from the bottom of the pan. Set aside until warm.

5. When the dough is warm, knead, adding the remaining flour until it is smooth and elastic.

6. Roll the dough into a floured surface.

7. The format in circular portions.

8. Stuff with the shrimp and arrange a spoonful of curd. Close by tightening the ends.

9. Dip into beaten egg, breadcrumbs, and fry in hot oil until golden brown.

Nutrition: Calories: 736 kcal Protein: 42.45 g Fat: 26.71 g Carbohydrates: 78.58 g

24. **Pumpkin Shrimp**

Difficulty level: Medium

Preparation time: 20 minutes

Cooking Time: 1 hour and 10 minutes

Servings: 4-6

Ingredients:

- 1 average pumpkin

- 1kg medium shrimp

- 1 white onion

- 3 cloves of garlic

- 2 cans of peeled tomatoes

- 1 cup of white wine

- 1 box of sour cream

- 1 cup of curd

- salt

- Aluminum paper

Directions:

1. Cut the lid off the pumpkin, wrap in foil and bake at 180 degrees for 15 minutes.

2. Remove from oven, remove seeds and return to oven for another 40 minutes at 180 degrees.

3. In a pan, sauté the chopped onion. When golden, add the garlic and sauté until the aroma is released.

4. Add the peeled tomato cans and the white wine. Cook for 15 minutes over medium heat. Add water if it dries too fast.

5. When the tomato is already well crushed, add the cream and 1/2 cup of curd. Let reduce until thickened — season with salt.

6. In a skillet with olive oil, cook the prawns over high heat. When they are golden, add to the sauce. Remove the pumpkin from the oven, pass the remaining cream cheese on the inner walls, and place the shrimp sauce inside.

Nutrition: Calories: 218 kcal Protein: 29.55 g Fat: 5.94 g Carbohydrates: 10.65 g

25. **Tiger Prawn Paella**

Difficulty level: Hard

Preparation time: 10 minutes

Cooking Time: 25 minutes

Servings: 4

Ingredients:

- 1 lb. tiger prawns, whole

- 2 cups cauliflower, chopped into florets

- 1 small red bell pepper, finely chopped

- 4 cups fish stock

- 1 tsp apple cider vinegar

- 2 small onion, finely chopped

- 3 garlic cloves, crushed

- 5 bacon slices, chopped

- 3 tbsp. butter

- Spices:

- 4 tbsp. fresh parsley, finely chopped

- 1 tsp sea salt

- ½ tsp black pepper, freshly ground

- 2 tsp turmeric powder

- ½ tsp saffron threads

Directions:

1. Set the instant pot then put cauliflower. Put in the fish stock and sprinkle with salt. Close the lid and set the steam release handle to the "Sealing" position. Press the "Manual" button then set the timer for 5 minutes on high pressure.

2. Once done, perform a quick release and open the lid. Take off the cauliflower from the pot and drain. Make sure to reserve the stock. Set aside.

3. Press the "Sauté" button then grease the inner pot with butter. Heat up then add onions and garlic. Stir-fry for 4-5 minutes.

4. Put bell pepper and bacon. Cook and stir for 3-4 more minutes. Season with some more salt, pepper, and turmeric powder.

5. Stir well and add prawns and cauliflower. Put in the remaining stock and close the lid.

6. Set the steam release handle again and press the "Manual" button. Set the timer for at least 8 minutes on high pressure.

7. Once done, release the pressure and open the lid. Mix well and sprinkle with saffron and fresh parsley. Allow it to sit for a while before serving.

8. Optionally, press the "Sauté" button again and simmer until all the liquid evaporates.

Nutrition: Calories 419 Total Fats 22.6g Net Carbs: 8.5g Protein: 41.8g Fiber: 2.5g

CHAPTER 4:

POULTRY

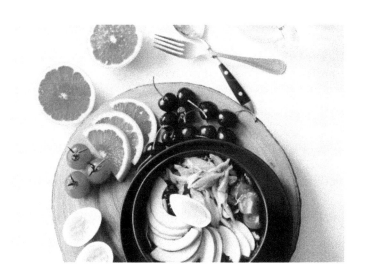

26. <u>Almond Chicken Cutlets</u>

Difficulty level: Easy

Preparation time: 10 minutes

Cooking Time: 15 minutes

Servings: 4

Ingredients:

- 2 eggs

- ½ teaspoon garlic powder

- 1 cup almond flour

- 1 tablespoon chopped fresh oregano

- 4 (4-ounce) boneless skinless chicken breasts, pounded to about ¼ inch thick

- ¼ cup good-quality olive oil

- 2 tablespoons grass-fed butter

Directions:

1. Bread the chicken. Whisk together the eggs, garlic powder in a medium bowl, and set it aside. Stir together the almond flour and oregano on a plate and set the plate next to the egg mixture. Pat the chicken breasts to dry using paper towels and dip them into the egg mixture. Remove excess egg then roll the chicken in the almond flour until they are coated.

2. Fry the chicken. In a large skillet over medium-high heat, warm the olive oil and butter. Add the breaded chicken breasts and

fry them, turning them once, until they are cooked through, very crispy, and golden brown, and 14 to 16 minutes in total.

3. Serve. Place one cutlet on each of four plates and serve them immediately.

Nutrition: Calories: 328 Total fat: 23g Total carbs: 0g Fiber: 0g Net carbs: 0g Sodium: 75mg Protein: 28g

27. **Slow Cooker Chicken Cacciatore**

Difficulty level: Easy Preparation time: 15 minutes

Cooking Time: 10 minutes   Servings: 4

Ingredients:

- ¼ cup good-quality olive oil

- 4 (4-ounce) boneless chicken breasts, each cut into three pieces

- 1 onion, chopped 2 celery stalks, chopped

- 1 cup sliced mushrooms

- 2 tablespoons minced garlic

- 1 (28-ounce) can sodium-free diced tomatoes

- ½ cup red wine

- ½ cup tomato paste

- 1 tablespoon dried basil

- 1 teaspoon dried oregano

- ⅛ teaspoon red pepper flakes

Directions:

1. Brown the chicken. In a skillet at medium-high heat, warm the olive oil. Add the chicken breasts and brown them, turning them once, about 10 minutes in total.

2. Cook in the slow cooker. Place the chicken in the slow cooker and stir in the onion, celery, mushrooms, garlic, tomatoes, red wine, tomato paste, basil, oregano, and red pepper flakes. Cook it on high for approximately 3 to 4 hours or on low for 6 to 8 hours, until the chicken is fully cooked and tender.

3. Serve. Divide the chicken and sauce between four bowls and serve it immediately.

Nutrition: Calories: 383 Total fat: 26g Total carbs: 11g Fiber: 4g Net carbs: 7g Sodium: 116mg Protein: 26g

28. <u>Cheesy Chicken Sun-Dried Tomato</u>

<u>Packets</u>

Difficulty level: Easy

Preparation time: 15 minutes

Cooking Time: 40 minutes

Servings: 4

Ingredients:

- 1 cup goat cheese

- ½ cup chopped oil-packed sun-dried tomatoes

- 1 teaspoon minced garlic

- ½ teaspoon dried basil

- ½ teaspoon dried oregano

- 4 (4-ounce) boneless chicken breasts

- Sea salt, for seasoning

- Freshly ground black pepper, for seasoning

- 3 tablespoons olive oil

Directions:

1. Preheat the oven. Set the oven temperature to 375°F.

2. Prepare the filling. In a medium bowl, put the goat cheese, sun-dried tomatoes, garlic, basil, and oregano then mix until everything is well blended.

3. Stuff the chicken. Make a horizontal slice in the middle of each chicken breast to make a pocket, making sure not to cut through the sides or ends. Spoon one-quarter of the filling into each breast, folding the skin and chicken meat over the slit to form packets. Secure the packets with a toothpick. Lightly season the breasts with salt and pepper.

4. Brown the chicken. In a large oven-safe skillet over medium heat, warm the olive oil. Add the breasts and sear them, turning them once, until they are golden, about 8 minutes in total.

5. Bake the chicken. Bring the skillet into the oven and bake the chicken for 30 minutes or until it's cooked through.

6. Serve. Remove the toothpicks. Divide the chicken into 4 plates and serve them immediately.

Nutrition: Calories: 388 Total fat: 29g Total carbs: 4g Fiber: 1g; Net carbs: 3g Sodium: 210mg Protein: 28g

29. **Tuscan Chicken Saute**

Difficulty level: Easy Preparation time: 10 minutes

Cooking Time: 35 minutes Servings: 4

Ingredients:

- 1 pound boneless chicken breasts, each cut into three pieces

- Sea salt, for seasoning

- Freshly ground black pepper, for seasoning

- 3 tablespoons olive oil

- 1 tablespoon minced garlic

- ¾ cup chicken stock

- 1 teaspoon dried oregano

- ½ teaspoon dried basil

- ½ cup heavy (whipping) cream

- ½ cup shredded Asiago cheese

- 1 cup fresh spinach

- ¼ cup sliced Kalamata olives

Directions:

1. Prepare the chicken. Pat, the chicken, breasts dry and lightly season them with salt and pepper.

2. Sauté the chicken. In a large skillet over medium-high heat, warm the olive oil. Add the chicken and sauté until it is golden brown and just cooked through, about 15 minutes in total. Transfer the chicken to a plate and set it aside.

3. Make the sauce. Put the garlic to the skillet, then sauté until it's softened about 2 minutes. Stir in the chicken stock, oregano, and basil, scraping up any browned bits in the skillet. Bring to a boil, then reduce the heat to low and simmer until the sauce is reduced by about one-quarter, about 10 minutes.

4. Finish the dish. Stir in the cream, Asiago, and simmer, stirring the sauce frequently, until it has thickened about 5 minutes. Put back the chicken to the skillet along with any accumulated juices. Stir in the spinach and olives and simmer until the spinach is wilted about 2 minutes.

5. Serve. Divide the chicken and sauce between four plates and serve it immediately.

Nutrition: Calories: 483 Total fat: 38g Total carbs: 5g Fiber: 1g; Net carbs: 3g Sodium: 332mg Protein: 31g

30. **Breaded Chicken Fillets**

Difficulty level: Easy

Preparation time: 5 minutes

Cooking Time: 10-25 minutes

Servings: 4

Ingredients:

- 1 pound chicken fillets

- 3 bell peppers, quartered lengthwise

- 1/3 cup Romano cheese

- 2 teaspoons olive oil

- 1 garlic clove, minced

- Kosher salt, to taste

- Ground black pepper, to taste

- 1/3 cup crushed pork rinds

Directions:

1. Set oven to 410°F

2. Mix the crushed pork rinds, Romano cheese, olive oil, and minced garlic. Dredge the chicken into this mixture.

3. Bring the chicken into a lightly greased baking sheet. Sprinkle with salt and black pepper to taste.

4. Scatter the peppers around the chicken and bake in the preheated oven for 20 to 25 minutes or until thoroughly cooked.

Nutrition: 367 Calories 16.9g Fat 6g Carbs 43g Protein 0.7g Fiber

31. **Turkey Ham and Mozzarella Pate**

Difficulty level: Easy

Preparation time: 10 minutes

Cooking Time: 0 minutes

Servings: 6

Ingredients:

- 4 ounces turkey ham, chopped

- 2 tablespoons fresh parsley, roughly chopped

- 2 tablespoons flaxseed meal

- 4 ounces mozzarella cheese, crumbled

- 2 tablespoons sunflower seeds

Directions:

1. Thoroughly combine the ingredients, except for the sunflower seeds, in your food processor.

2. Spoon the mixture into a serving bowl and scatter the sunflower seeds over the top.

Nutrition: 212 Calories 18.8g Fat 2g Carbs 10.6g Protein 1.6g Fiber

32. <u>**Boozy Glazed Chicken**</u>

Difficulty level: Easy

Preparation time: 5 minutes

Cooking Time: 55 minutes

Servings: 4

Ingredients:

- 2 pounds chicken drumettes

- 2 tablespoons ghee, at room temperature

- Sea salt, to taste

- Ground black pepper, to taste

- 1 teaspoon Mediterranean seasoning mix

- 2 vine-ripened tomatoes, pureed

- 3/4 cup rum

- 3 tablespoons coconut aminos

- A few drops of liquid Stevia

- 1 teaspoon chile peppers, minced

- 1 tablespoon minced fresh ginger

- 1 teaspoon ground cardamom

- 2 tablespoons fresh lemon juice, + wedges for serving

Directions:

1. Toss the chicken with the melted ghee, salt, black pepper, and Mediterranean seasoning mix until well coated on all sides.

2. In another bowl, thoroughly combine the pureed tomato puree, rum, coconut aminos, Stevia, chile peppers, ginger, cardamom, and lemon juice.

3. Pour the tomato mixture over the chicken drumettes; let it marinate for 2 hours. Bake in the preheated oven at 410 degrees F for about 45 minutes.

4. Add in the reserved marinade and place under the preheated broiler for 10 minutes.

Nutrition: 307 Calories 12.1g Fat 2.7g Carbs 33.6g Protein 1.5g Fiber

33. <u>Pan-Fried Chorizo Sausage</u>

Difficulty level: Easy Preparation time: 5 minutes

Cooking Time: 15 minutes Servings: 4

Ingredients:

- 16 ounces smoked turkey chorizo 1 ½ cups Asiago cheese, grated 1 teaspoon oregano

- 1 teaspoon basil - 1 cup tomato puree

- 4 scallion stalks, chopped 1 teaspoon garlic paste

- Sea salt, to taste Ground black pepper, to taste

- 1 tablespoon dry sherry 1 tablespoon extra-virgin olive oil

- 2 tablespoons fresh coriander, roughly chopped

Directions:

1. In a skillet, put oil and heat it over moderately high heat. Now, brown the turkey chorizo, crumbling with a fork for about 5 minutes.

2. Add in the other ingredients, except for cheese; continue to cook for 10 minutes more or until cooked through.

Nutrition: 330 Calories17.2g Fat 4.5g Carbs 34.4g Protein 1.6g Fiber

34. **Easy Chicken Tacos**

Difficulty level: Easy

Preparation time: 5 minutes

Cooking Time: 27 minutes

Servings: 4

Ingredients:

- 1 pound ground chicken

- 1 ½ cups Mexican cheese blend

- 1 tablespoon Mexican seasoning blend

- 2 teaspoons butter, room temperature

- 2 small-sized shallots, peeled and finely chopped

- 1 clove garlic, minced

- 1 cup tomato puree

- 1/2 cup salsa

- 2 slices bacon, chopped

Directions:

1. In a saucepan, put butter then melt in over a moderately high flame. Now, cook the shallots until tender and fragrant.

2. Then, sauté the garlic, chicken, and bacon for about 5 minutes, stirring continuously and crumbling with a fork. Add the in Mexican seasoning blend.

3. Fold in the tomato puree and salsa; continue to simmer for 5 to 7 minutes over medium-low heat; reserve.

4. Line a baking pan with wax paper. Place 4 piles of the shredded cheese on the baking pan and gently press them down with a wide spatula to make "taco shells."

5. Bake in the preheated oven at 365 degrees F for 6 to 7 minutes or until melted. Allow these taco shells to cool for about 10 minutes.

Nutrition: 535 Calories33.3g Fat .8g Carbs 47.9g Protein 1.9g Fiber

35. <u>**Cheesy Bacon-Wrapped Chicken with Asparagus Spears**</u>

Difficulty level: Medium

Preparation time: 20 minutes

Cooking Time: 30 minutes

Servings: 4

Ingredients:

- 4 chicken breasts

- 8 bacon slices

- 1 pound (454 g) asparagus spears

- 2 tablespoons fresh lemon juice

- ½ cup Manchego cheese, grated

- From the cupboard

- 4 tablespoons olive oil, divided

- Salt, to taste

- Freshly ground black pepper, to taste

Directions:

1. Set the oven to 400°F. Line a baking sheet using parchment paper, then grease with 1 tablespoon olive oil.

2. Put the chicken breasts in a large bowl, and sprinkle with salt and black pepper. Toss to combine well.

3. Wrap every chicken breast with 2 slices of bacon. Place the chicken on the baking sheet, then bake in the preheated oven for 25 minutes or until the bacon is crispy.

4. Preheat the grill to high, then brush with the remaining olive oil.

5. Place the asparagus spears on the grill grate, and sprinkle with salt. Grill for 5 minutes or until fork-tender. Flip the asparagus frequently during the grilling.

6. Transfer the bacon-wrapped chicken breasts to four plates, drizzle with lemon juice, and scatter with Manchego cheese. Spread the hot asparagus spears on top to serve.

Nutrition: Calories: 455 Total fat: 38.1g Net carbs: 2g Protein: 26.1g

36. **Bacon-Wrapped Chicken with Cheddar Cheese**

Difficulty level: Medium

Preparation time: 10 minutes

Cooking Time:

4 hours

Servings: 6

Ingredients:

- 2 large chicken breasts, each cut into 6 pieces

- 6 slices of streaky bacon, each cut in half widthways

- 4 garlic cloves, crushed

- ½ cup Cheddar cheese, grated

- From the cupboard:

- 1 tablespoon olive oil

- Salt, to taste

- Freshly ground black pepper, to taste

Directions:

1. Grease the insert of the slow cooker with olive oil.

2. Wrap each piece of chicken breast with each half of the bacon slice, and arrange them in the slow cooker. Sprinkle with garlic, salt, and black pepper.

3. Put the lid and then cook on LOW for 4 hours.

4. Set the oven to 350°F (180°C).

5. Transfer the cooked bacon-wrapped chicken to a baking dish, then scatter with cheese.

6. Cook in the preheated oven for 5 minutes or until the cheese melts.

7. Take it off from the oven and serve warm.

Nutrition: Calories: 308 Total fat: 20.8g Total carbs: 2.9g Fiber: 0g Net carbs: 2.9g Protein: 26.1g

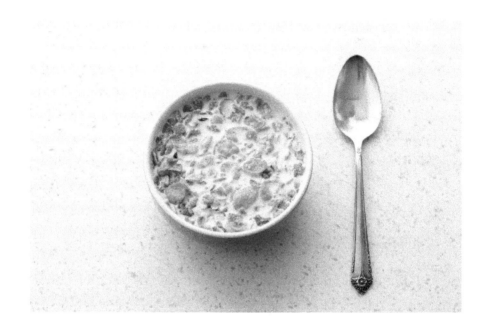

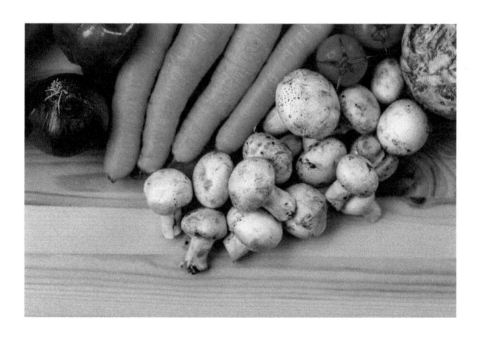

CHAPTER 5:

MEAT

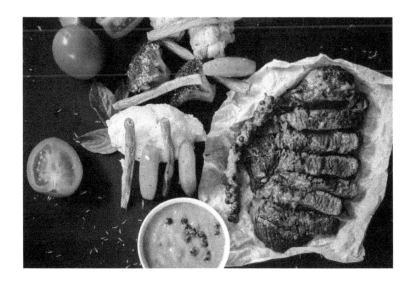

37. <u>Chili Beef and Beans</u>

Difficulty level: Medium

Preparation time: 10 minutes

Cooking Time: 10 minutes

Servings: 5-6

Ingredients:

- ounces beef, finely chopped

- 4 carrots, chopped

- 2 onions, chopped

- 1 can (14 ounces) diced tomatoes

- 2 cans (14 ounces each) mixed beans, drained

- 1 teaspoon garam masala

- 2 teaspoons cumin powder

- 2 teaspoons chili paste or sambal oelek

- Oil, to cook

- ½ cup water

- Cooked brown rice to serve

Directions:

1. Place a pan over high heat. Add a little oil. When the oil is heated, add 1 teaspoon chili powder, beef, and 1 teaspoon cumin powder, and sauté for a couple of minutes. Transfer into a bowl.

2. Put a bit of oil into the same pan. When the oil is heated, add carrots and onion and sauté until onions are light brown.

3. Add the rest of the ingredients and mix well. Cook for 3-5 minutes. Add some water if you find the chili very thick.

4. Add beef into the pan and mix well. Heat for 3-5 minutes.

5. Place brown rice in serving bowls. Ladle chili on top and serve.

Nutrition: Calories: 149 kcal Protein: 13.04 g Fat: 4.99 g Carbohydrates: 14.27 g

38. <u>Mustard Lamb Lunch</u>

Difficulty level: Medium

Preparation time: 10 minutes

Cooking Time: 35 minutes

Servings: 4

Ingredients:

- 2 (8-rib) lamb racks, patted dry

- ¼ cup Dijon mustard

- 2 tablespoons chopped fresh thyme

- 1 tablespoon chopped fresh rosemary

- Freshly ground black pepper, to taste

- Salt, to taste

- 1 tablespoon olive oil

Directions:

1. Preheat an oven to 425°F.

2. In a mixing bowl, put together the mustard, thyme, and rosemary then mix.

3. Coat the lamb racks with sea salt and pepper.

4. Place a large ovenproof skillet over the medium-high cooking flame and heat the olive oil.

5. Add the lamb rack; stir-cook for about 2 minutes per side, turning once.

6. Take it out from the heat and top with the mustard mix.

7. Bake for 30 minutes or until cooks well.

8. Remove the lamb racks and cut them into pieces. Serve warm.

Nutrition: Calories 413 Fat 24g Carbohydrates 2g Fiber 1g Protein 52g

39. **Apple Pork Raisins**

Difficulty level: Medium

Preparation time: 10 minutes

Cooking Time: 30 minutes

Servings: 4

Ingredients:

- Salsa:

- ½ teaspoon (shredded or grated) fresh ginger

- 2 apples, peeled, cored, and diced

- 1 teaspoon olive oil

- ¼ cup finely chopped sweet onion

- ½ cup dried raisins

- Pinch sea salt

- Chops:

- 4 (4-ounce) boneless center-cut pork chops, trimmed and patted dry

- Freshly ground black pepper, to taste

- Salt to taste

- 1 teaspoon garlic powder

- 1 teaspoon ground cinnamon

- 1 tablespoon olive oil

Directions:

1. In a skillet or saucepan, warm the oil on the medium stove flame.

2. Add the onions, ginger, stir the mixture and cook while stirring for about 2-3 minutes until softened.

3. Stir in the apples and raisins. Sauté for about 4-5 minutes.

4. Season with sea salt and set it aside.

5. Coat the pork chops each side with the garlic powder, cinnamon, sea salt, and pepper.

6. In a skillet or saucepan, warm the oil on the medium stove flame.

7. Add the chops and cook, while stirring, until it becomes evenly brown.

8. Serve the chops with the apple salsa.

Nutrition: Calories 384 Fat 27g Carbohydrates 11g Fiber 2g Protein 26g

40. **Avocado Pineapple Pork**

Difficulty level: Medium Preparation time: 10 minutes

Cooking Time: 40 minutes

Servings: 4

Ingredients:

- 1 teaspoon cumin

- 8 ounces canned pineapple, crushed

- 1 tablespoon olive oil

- 1 pound pork, ground

- 1 teaspoon chili powder

- 1 teaspoon garlic powder

- (ground) black pepper and salt to taste

- 1 mango, chopped

- Juice of 1 lime

- 2 avocados, pitted, peeled and chopped

- ¼ cup cilantro, chopped

Directions:

1. In a skillet or saucepan, warm the oil on the medium stove flame.

2. Put the pork and cook, while stirring, until it becomes evenly brown.

3. Add the garlic, cumin, chili powder, salt and pepper, stir cook for 7-8 minutes.

4. Add the pineapple, mango, avocados, lime juice, cilantro, salt, and pepper; stir-cook for 5-6 minutes.

5. Divide between serving plates and serve.

Nutrition: Calories 238 Fat 6g Carbohydrates 12g Fiber 7g Protein 17g

41. <u>**Berry Chops Dinner**</u>

Difficulty level: Medium

Preparation time: 10 minutes

Cooking Time: 15 minutes

Servings: 4

Ingredients:

- 2 pounds pork chops

- ½ teaspoon thyme, dried

- 2 tablespoons water

- 1 teaspoon cinnamon powder

- (ground) black pepper and salt to taste

- 12 ounces blackberries

- ½ cup balsamic vinegar

Directions:

1. Spice the pork chops with salt, pepper, cinnamon, and thyme.

2. Heat up a cooking pot; add the blackberries and heat over medium heat.

3. Add the vinegar, water, salt, and pepper, stir the mix.

4. Simmer for 3-5 minutes and take it off the heat.

5. Brush the pork chops with half of the blueberry mix.

6. Preheat your grill and grill the chops over medium heat for 6 minutes on each side.

7. Divide the pork chops between serving plates; top with the rest of the blackberry sauce. Serve warm.

Nutrition: Calories 286 Fat 6g Carbohydrates 11g Fiber 6g Protein 22g

42. **Cauliflower Lamb Meal**

Difficulty level: Medium Preparation time: 5 minutes

Cooking Time: 20 minutes

Servings: 4

Ingredients:

- Mash:

- 1 large head cauliflower, cut into florets

- ½ teaspoon garlic powder

- ½ teaspoon salt

- Dash cayenne pepper

- Lamb:

- 2 (8-ounce) grass-fed lamb fillets

- 2 tablespoons avocado oil

- 1 teaspoon dried rosemary

- 1 teaspoon salt

- ½ teaspoon freshly ground black pepper

Directions:

1. In cooking (you can also use a saucepan), add the cauliflower and water to cover it.

2. Heat it over the medium stove flame. Boil and cook for 10 minutes. Drain water and transfer the cauliflower to a food processor (or blender).

3. Add the ghee, garlic powder, salt, and cayenne pepper. Blend to a smooth consistency.

4. Spice the lamb with the pepper and salt.

5. In a skillet or saucepan, warm the oil on the medium stove flame.

6. Add the lamb, rosemary, and cook, while stirring, until it becomes evenly brown for 8-10 minutes.

7. Slice the lamb into coins and serve with the cauliflower mash.

Nutrition: Calories 294 Fat 17g Carbohydrates 11g Fiber 3g Protein 36g

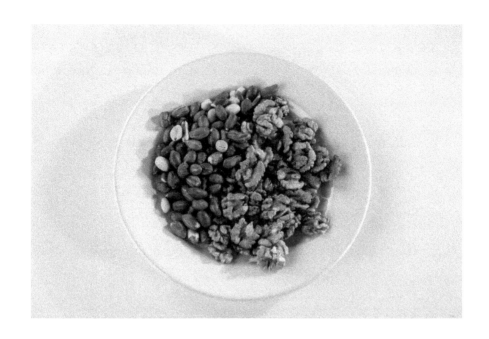

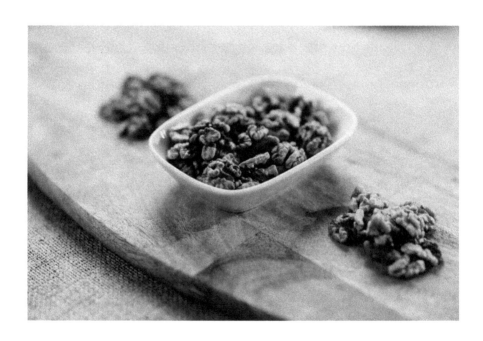

CHAPTER 6:

SNACKS

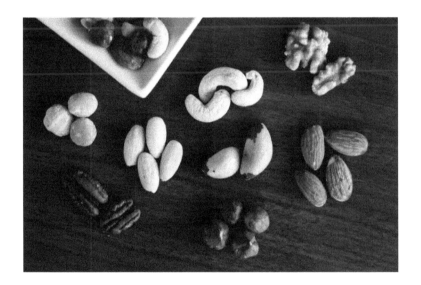

43. **Tangy Turmeric Flavored Florets**

Difficulty level: Medium

Preparation time: 10 minutes

Cooking Time: 55 minutes

Servings: 1

Ingredients:

- 1-head cauliflower, chopped into florets

- 1-Tbsp olive oil

- 1-Tbsp turmeric

- A pinch of cumin

- A dash of salt

Directions:

1. Set the oven to 400°F.

2. Put all together the ingredients in a baking pan. Mix well until thoroughly combined.

3. Cover the pan with foil. Roast for 40 minutes. Remove the foil cover and roast additionally for 15 minutes.

Nutrition: Calories: 90 Fat: 3g Protein: 4.5g Sodium: 87mg Total Carbs: 16.2g Dietary Fiber: 5g Net Carbs: 11.2g

CHAPTER 7:

DESSERTS

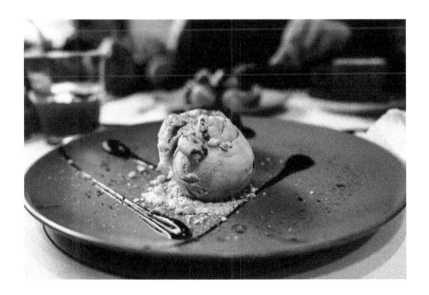

44. <u>Pistachioed Panna-Cotta Cocoa</u>

Difficulty level: Easy

Preparation time: 18 minutes

Cooking Time: 2 minutes

Servings: 6

Ingredients:

- 12-oz. dark chocolate

- 1-Tbsp coconut oil

- 3-pcs large bananas, sliced into thirds

- Cocoa nibs, chopped

- Spiced or smoked almonds, chopped

- Salted pistachios, chopped

Directions:

1. Line a baking pan with parchment paper.

2. Melt the dark chocolate with oil in your microwave. Set aside.

3. Pierce a Popsicle stick halfway into one end of each banana.

4. Dip each banana into the melted chocolate. Place dipped bananas into the baking sheet. Sprinkle generously with the cocoa nibs, almonds, and pistachios. Place the sheet in your freezer to harden and set.

Nutrition: Calories: 454 Fat: 15.1g Protein: 22.7g Sodium: 91mg Total Carbs: 61.6g Dietary Fiber: 4.9g Net Carbs: 56.7g

45. __Pure Avocado Pudding__

Difficulty level: Medium Preparation time: 3 hours

Cooking Time: 0 minutes Servings: 4

Ingredients:

- 1 cup almond milk

- 2 avocados, peeled and pitted

- ¾ cup cocoa powder

- 1 teaspoon vanilla extract

- 2 tablespoons stevia

- ¼ teaspoon cinnamon

- Walnuts, chopped for serving

Directions:

1. Add avocados to a blender and pulse well

2. Add cocoa powder, almond milk, stevia, vanilla bean extract and pulse the mixture well

3. Place into serving bowls then top with walnuts

4. Chill for 2-3 hours and serve!

Nutrition: Calories: 221 Fat: 8g Carbohydrates: 7g Protein: 3g

46. <u>Sweet Almond And Coconut Fat Bombs</u>

Difficulty level: Medium Preparation time: 10 minutes + 20 minutes chill time Cooking Time: 0 minutes Servings: 4

Ingredients:

- ¼ cup melted coconut oil

- 9 and ½ tablespoons almond butter

- 90 drops liquid stevia

- 3 tablespoons cocoa

- 9 tablespoons melted almond butter, sunflower seeds

Directions:

1. Take a bowl and add all of the listed ingredients

2. Mix them well

3. Pour scant 2 tablespoons of the mixture into as many muffin molds as you like

4. Chill for 20 minutes and pop them out

5. Serve and enjoy!

Nutrition: Total Carbs: 2g Fiber: 0g Protein: 2.53g Fat: 14g

47. <u>**Spicy Popper Mug Cake**</u>

Difficulty level: Medium

Preparation time: 5 minutes

Cooking Time: 5 minutes

Servings: 2

Ingredients:

- 2 tablespoons almond flour

- 1 tablespoon flaxseed meal

- 1 tablespoon almond butter

- 1 tablespoon cashew cheese

- 1 large egg

- 1 bacon, cooked and sliced

- ½ a jalapeno pepper

- ½ teaspoon baking powder

- ¼ teaspoon sunflower seeds

Directions:

1. Take a frying pan then place it on medium heat

2. Put sliced bacon and cook until they have a crispy texture

3. Take a microwave proof container and mix all of the listed ingredients(including cooked bacon), clean the sides

4. Microwave for 75 seconds making to put your microwave to high power

5. Take out the cup and slam it against a surface to take the cake out

6. Garnish with a bit of jalapeno and serve!

Nutrition: Calories: 429 Fat: 38g Carbohydrates: 6g Protein: 16g

48. The Most Elegant Parsley Soufflé Ever

Difficulty level: Medium Preparation time: 5 minutes

Cooking Time: 6 minutes Servings: 5

Ingredients:

- 2 whole eggs

- 1 fresh red chili pepper, chopped

- 2 tablespoons coconut cream

- 1 tablespoon fresh parsley, chopped

- Sunflower seeds to taste

Directions:

1. Preheat your oven to 390 degrees F

2. Almond butter 2 soufflé dishes

3. Put the ingredients to a blender and mix well

4. Divide batter into soufflé dishes and bake for 6 minutes

5. Serve and enjoy!

Nutrition: Calories: 108 Fat: 9g Carbohydrates: 9g Protein: 6g

49. __Fennel and Almond Bites__

Difficulty level: Medium Preparation time: 10 minutes + 3 hours freezing time Cooking Time: 25 minutes Servings: 10

Ingredients:

- 1 teaspoon vanilla extract

- ¼ cup almond milk

- ¼ cup of cocoa powder

- ½ cup almond oil

- A pinch of sunflower seeds

- 1 teaspoon fennel seeds

Directions:

1. Take a bowl and mix the almond oil and almond milk

2. Beat until smooth and glossy by using an electric beater

3. Mix in the rest of the ingredients

4. Take a piping bag and pour into a parchment paper-lined baking sheet

5. Freeze for 3 hours and stored in the fridge

Nutrition: Total Carbs: 1g Fiber: 1g Protein: 1g Fat: 20g

50. <u>Coconut Butter Fudge</u>

Difficulty level: Medium

Preparation time: 10 minutes

Cooking Time: 0 minutes

Servings: 6

Ingredients:

- 1 cup of coconut butter

- 2 tablespoons of raw honey

- ¼ teaspoon of salt

- 1 teaspoon of pure vanilla extract

Directions:

1. Begin by lining an 8 x 8 inch baking dish with parchment paper.

2. Melt the coconut butter, honey, and vanilla over low heat.

3. Put the mixture into the baking pan, and refrigerate for 2 hours before serving.

Nutrition: Total Carbohydrates: 6g Dietary Fiber: 0g Net Carbs: Protein: 0g Total Fat: 36g Calories: 334

CONCLUSION

If you've been suffering from chronic inflammation, it's likely you know already how difficult it can be to live with. From constant pain to unbearable itching, the side effects of this condition are enough to drive anyone mad. But what exactly is inflammation? And what if we told you that there are a number of different ways in which you can avoid the condition? You'd want to listen up then!

So, with that said, here are a few tips on how to avoid inflammation:

- Exercise regularly - Eat your greens - Drink plenty of fluids - Don't smoke

All these measures can help make your body stronger and healthier; decreasing your risk for developing chronic conditions such as inflammation.

1. Exercise regularly

Regular exercise keeps your muscles strong and supple, meaning that your joints and tissues are less likely to contract and swell up with inflammation. Stretching your body helps loosen the tendons, ligaments and muscles which can make you prone to inflammation when you're not using them.

2. Eat your greens

A large proportion of inflammation is caused by a build-up of toxins in the body; which means it's important that you get rid of all those pesky particles! Eating plenty of green veg will help clean out toxins, while helping keep your immune system strong. And speaking of immunity…

3. Drink plenty of fluids

A damaged 'immune system' can lead to over-reaction in the body, which is what leads to inflammation. So it's important that you remain hydrated throughout the day. Drinking lots of water will help keep your skin clear, while helping flush out toxins from the body! To learn more about how much water you need to drink per day, have a look at

Lightning Source UK Ltd.
Milton Keynes UK
UKHW020633280521
384530UK00001B/121